DIFFERENT COUSINS

by Marianne Reagan

AuthorHouse™
1663 Liberty Drive
Bloomington, IN 47403
www.authorhouse.com
Phone: 1-800-839-8640

First published by AuthorHouse 9/7/2011

ISBN: 978-1-4670-2508-9

Library of Congress Control Number: 2011915823

Printed in the United States of America
This book is printed on acid-free paper.

Any people depicted in stock imagery provided by Thinkstock are models,
and such images are being used for illustrative purposes only.
Certain stock imagery © Thinkstock.

Because of the dynamic nature of the Internet, any web addresses or links contained in this book may have changed
since publication and may no longer be valid. The views expressed in this work are solely those of the author and do not
necessarily reflect the views of the publisher, and the publisher hereby disclaims any responsibility for them.

Marianne Reagan lives at the Jersey shore with her husband John, son Johnny and daughter Kelly. She competes in
triathlons and combines her love of fitness with her passion for helping others collecting over $50,000 in donations for
various charities. You'll often find Marianne and Kelly at the mall making sure the aisles are accessible.

Illustrated by Mark "Gootz" Gutierrez is an illustrator, caricature artist and fine artist who has worked with a variety of clients. His work
has been featured in books, magazines, newspapers and television worldwide. He resides and works in Alexandria Virginia USA.

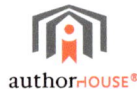

Foreword:

About 3,000 babies are born each year in the United States with cerebral palsy and approximately 300,000-500,000 people are affected with cerebral palsy in the United States. Cerebral means brain and palsy means there are issues with the way a person moves their body. A child with cerebral palsy may have problems controlling the muscles in their body. Depending on what part of the brain is affected, a child may have problems with one, two, three or all four limbs and may have difficulty communicating and learning. This story is about my daughter and how her type of cerebral palsy has affected her life.

Dedication:

To my beloved family who supports every endeavor I tackle and to my father who was the real writer in the family.

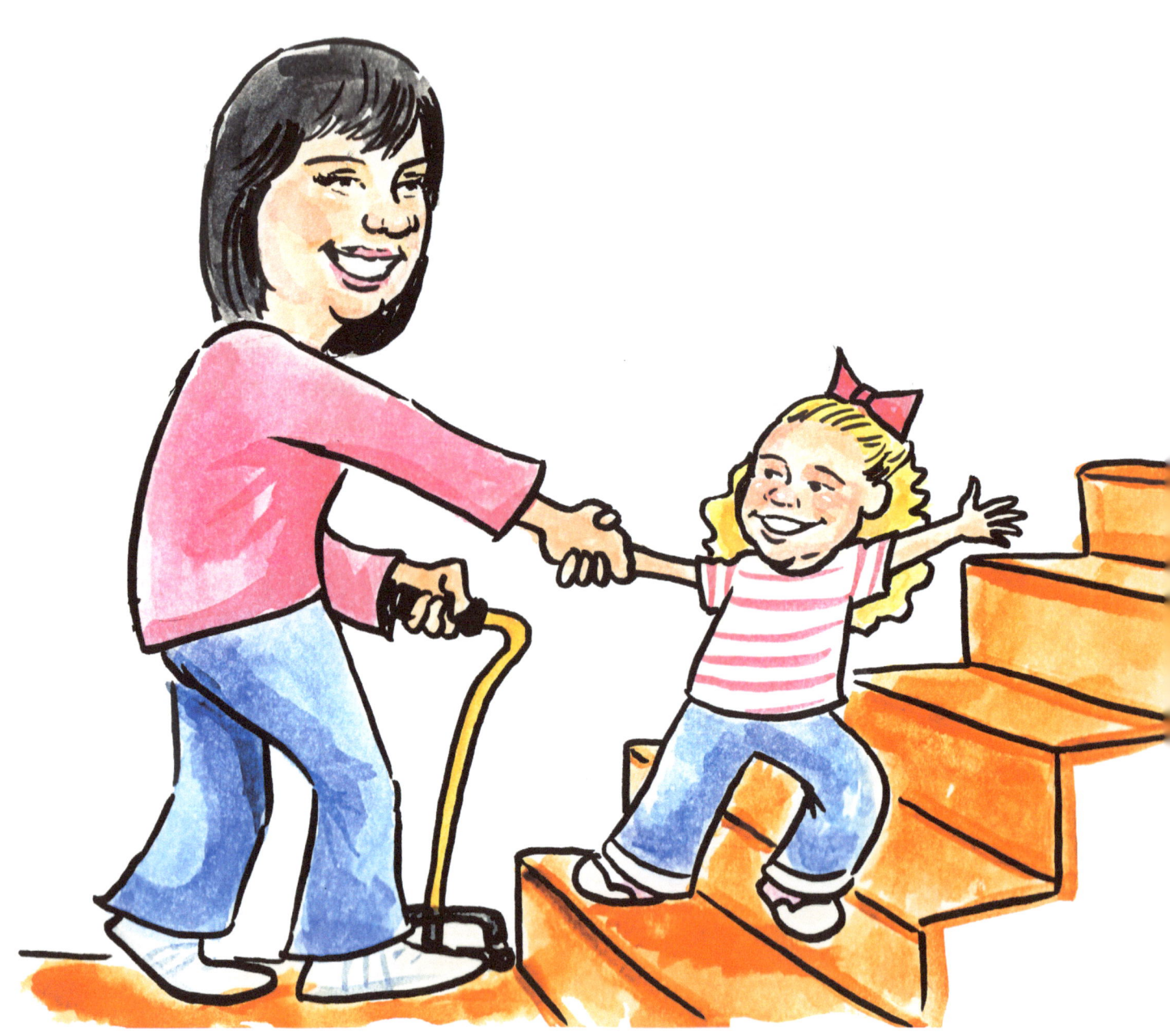

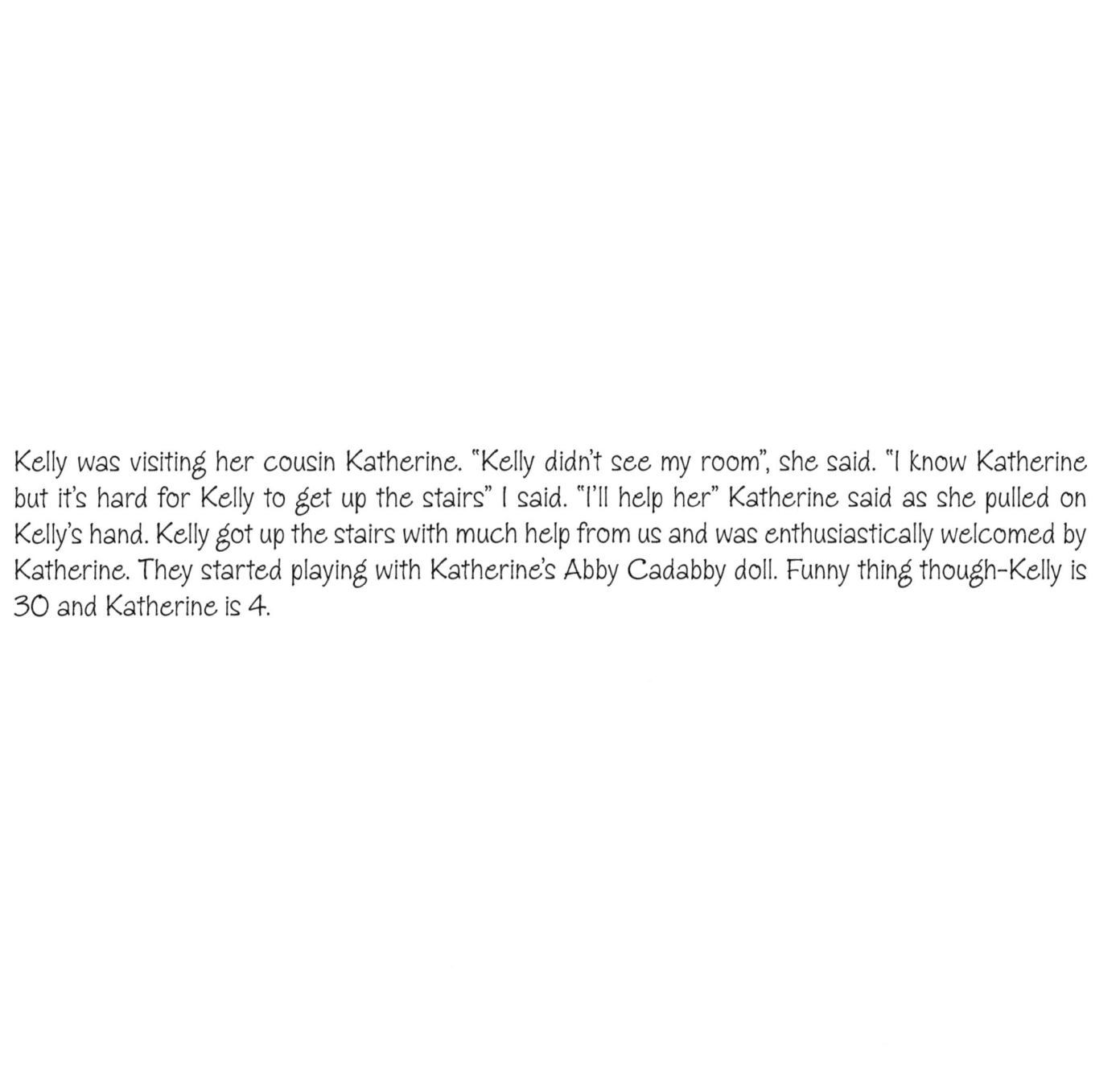

Kelly was visiting her cousin Katherine. "Kelly didn't see my room", she said. "I know Katherine but it's hard for Kelly to get up the stairs" I said. "I'll help her" Katherine said as she pulled on Kelly's hand. Kelly got up the stairs with much help from us and was enthusiastically welcomed by Katherine. They started playing with Katherine's Abby Cadabby doll. Funny thing though-Kelly is 30 and Katherine is 4.

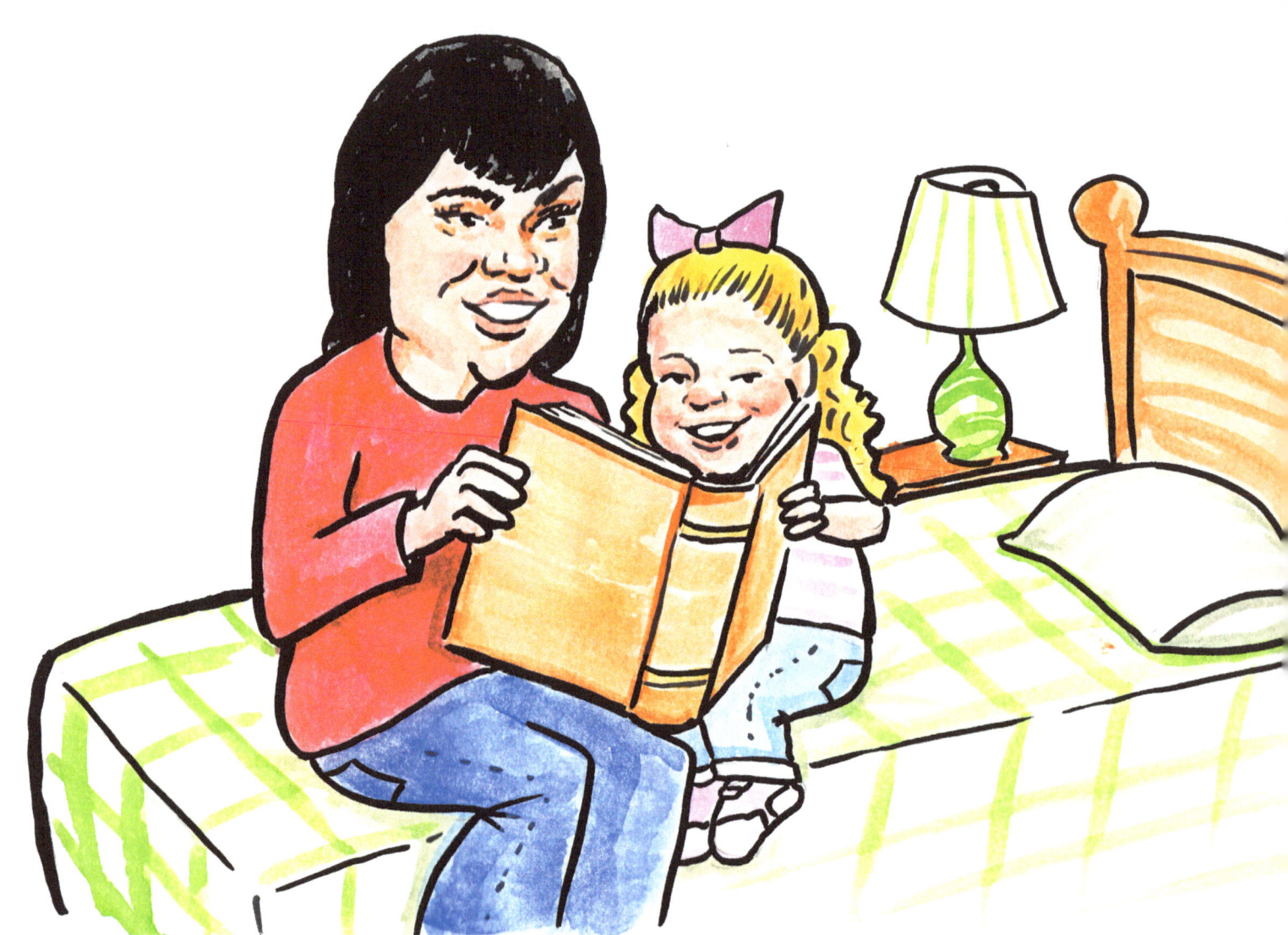

Kelly started reading a book to Katherine. Funny thing though–Kelly can't read and neither can Katherine yet.

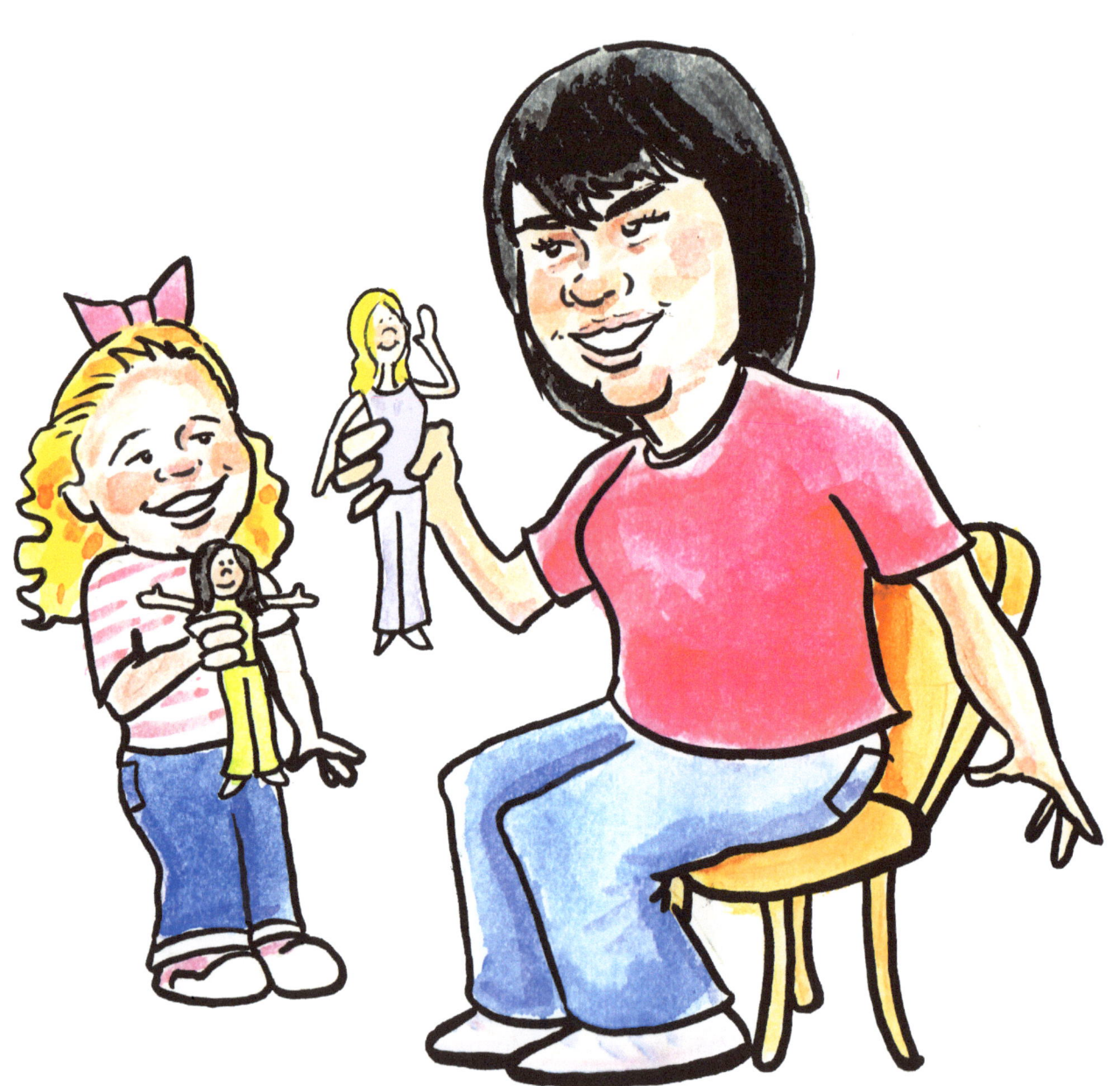

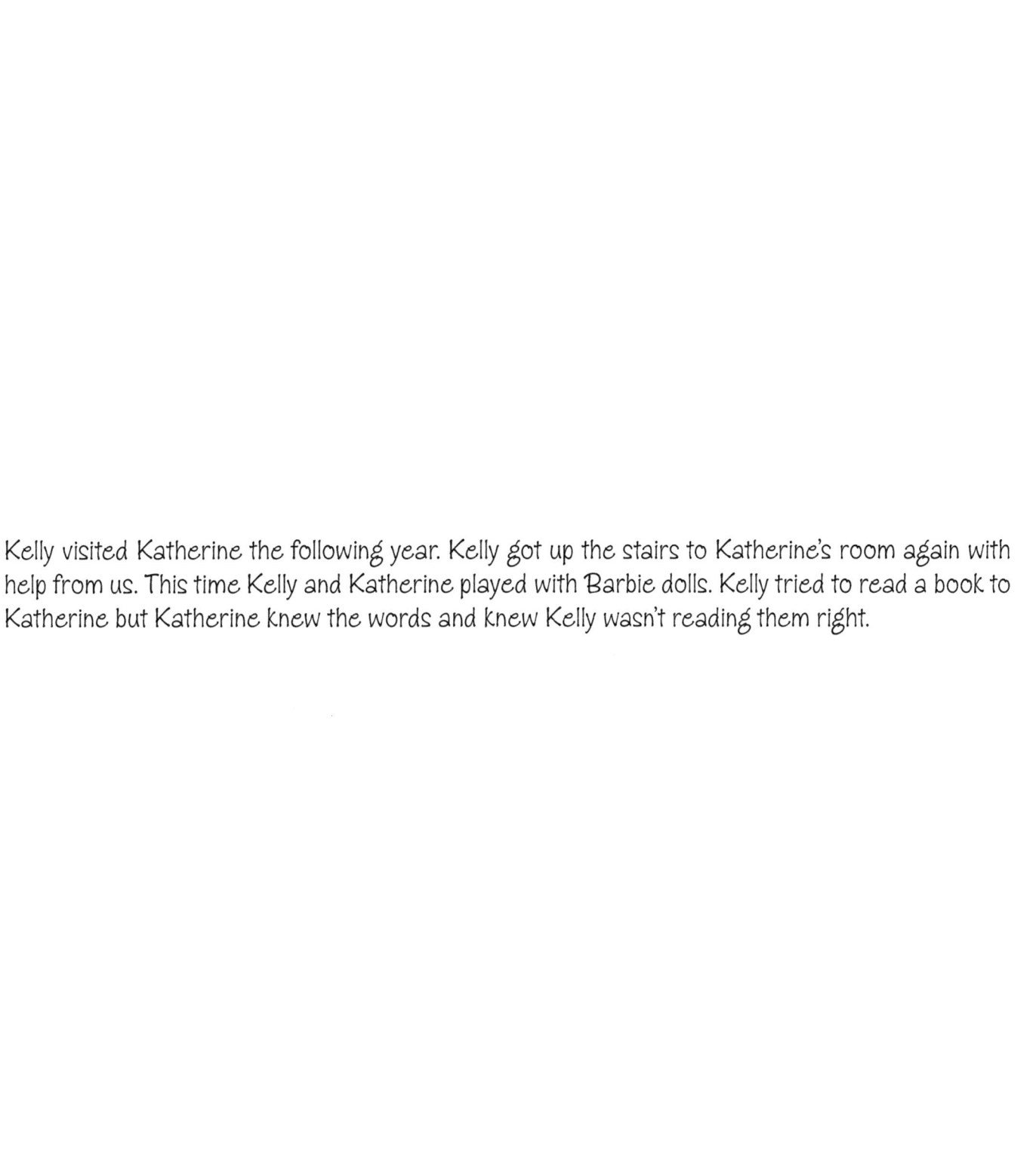

Kelly visited Katherine the following year. Kelly got up the stairs to Katherine's room again with help from us. This time Kelly and Katherine played with Barbie dolls. Kelly tried to read a book to Katherine but Katherine knew the words and knew Kelly wasn't reading them right.

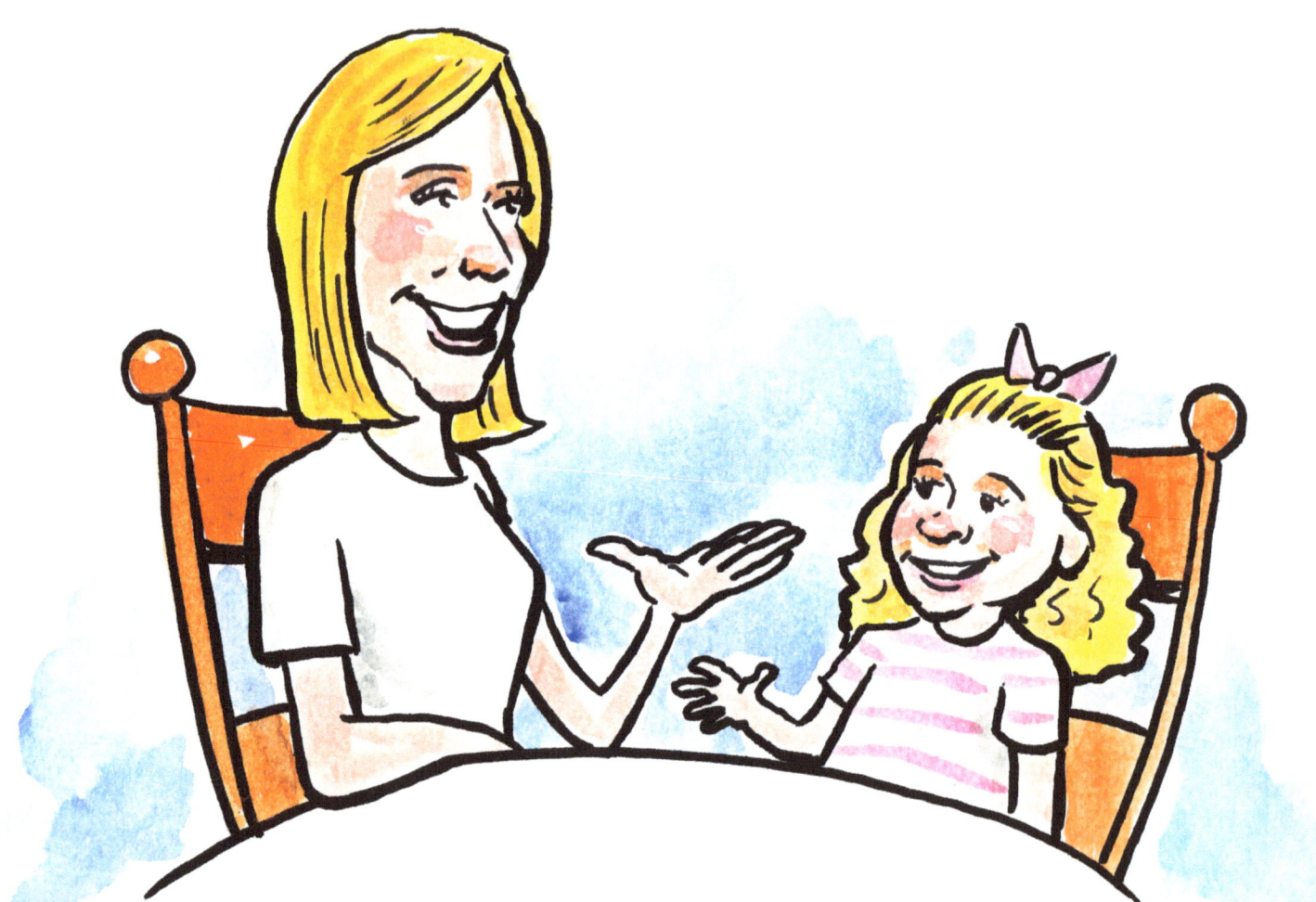

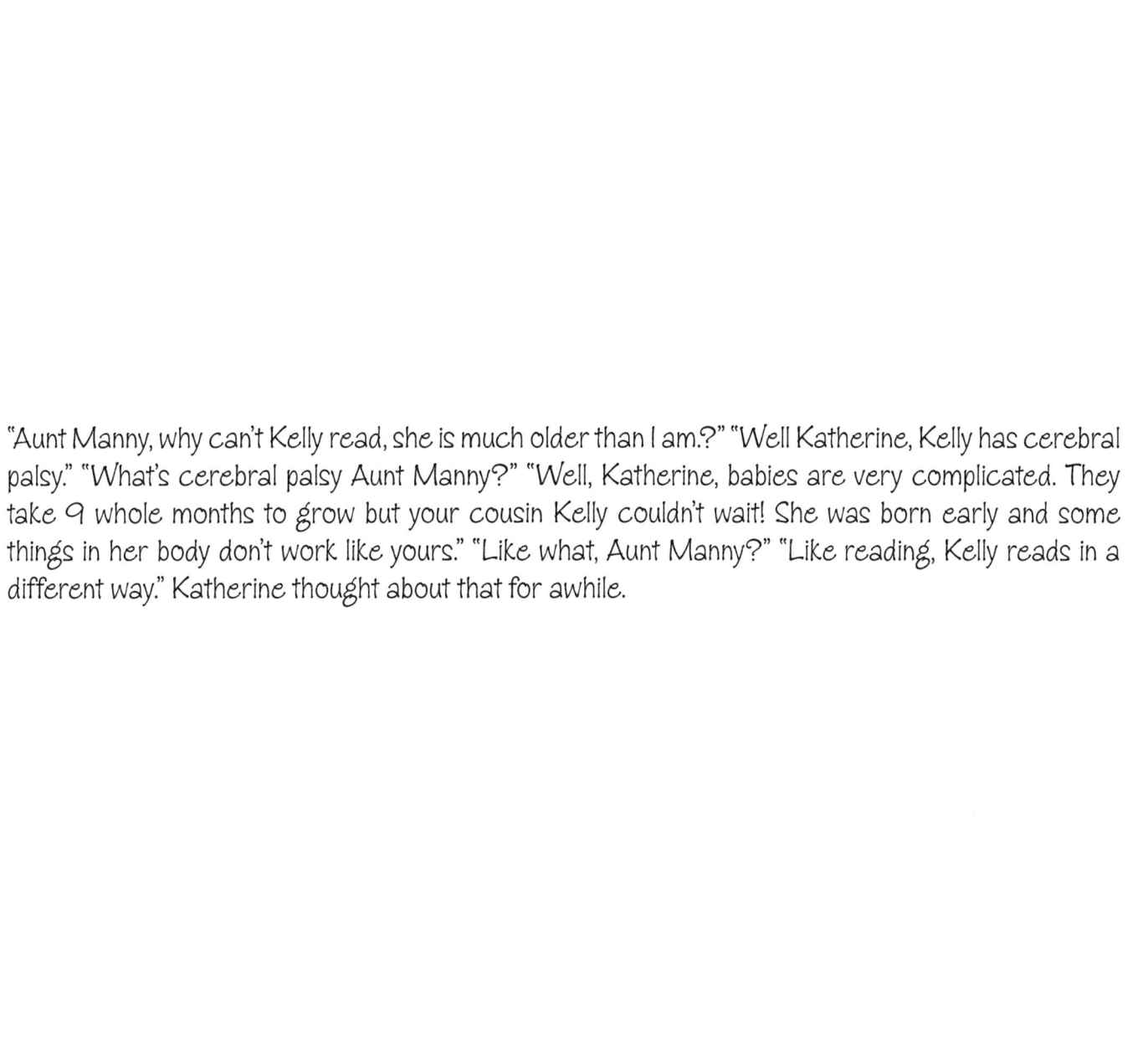

"Aunt Manny, why can't Kelly read, she is much older than I am.?" "Well Katherine, Kelly has cerebral palsy." "What's cerebral palsy Aunt Manny?" "Well, Katherine, babies are very complicated. They take 9 whole months to grow but your cousin Kelly couldn't wait! She was born early and some things in her body don't work like yours." "Like what, Aunt Manny?" "Like reading, Kelly reads in a different way." Katherine thought about that for awhile.

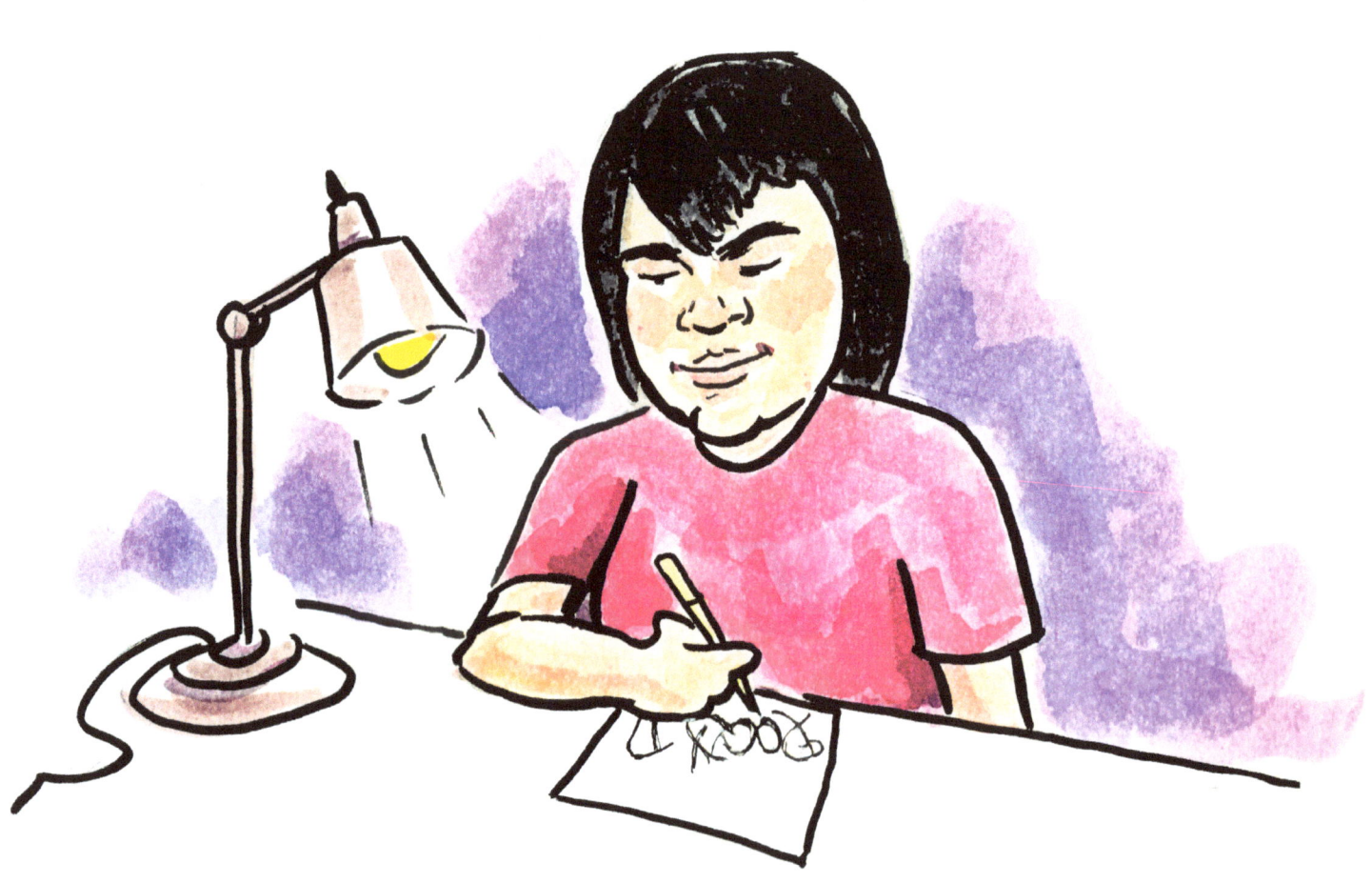

Katherine showed Kelly how she can write her name now. Kelly showed Katherine how she writes her name. "Aunt Manny, why does Kelly make scribbles for her name?" "Well Katherine, Kelly has cerebral palsy and learns in a different way. This is how Kelly writes her name." Katherine thought about that for awhile. And we thought about that. "Katherine, would you like to see what Kelly can do?"

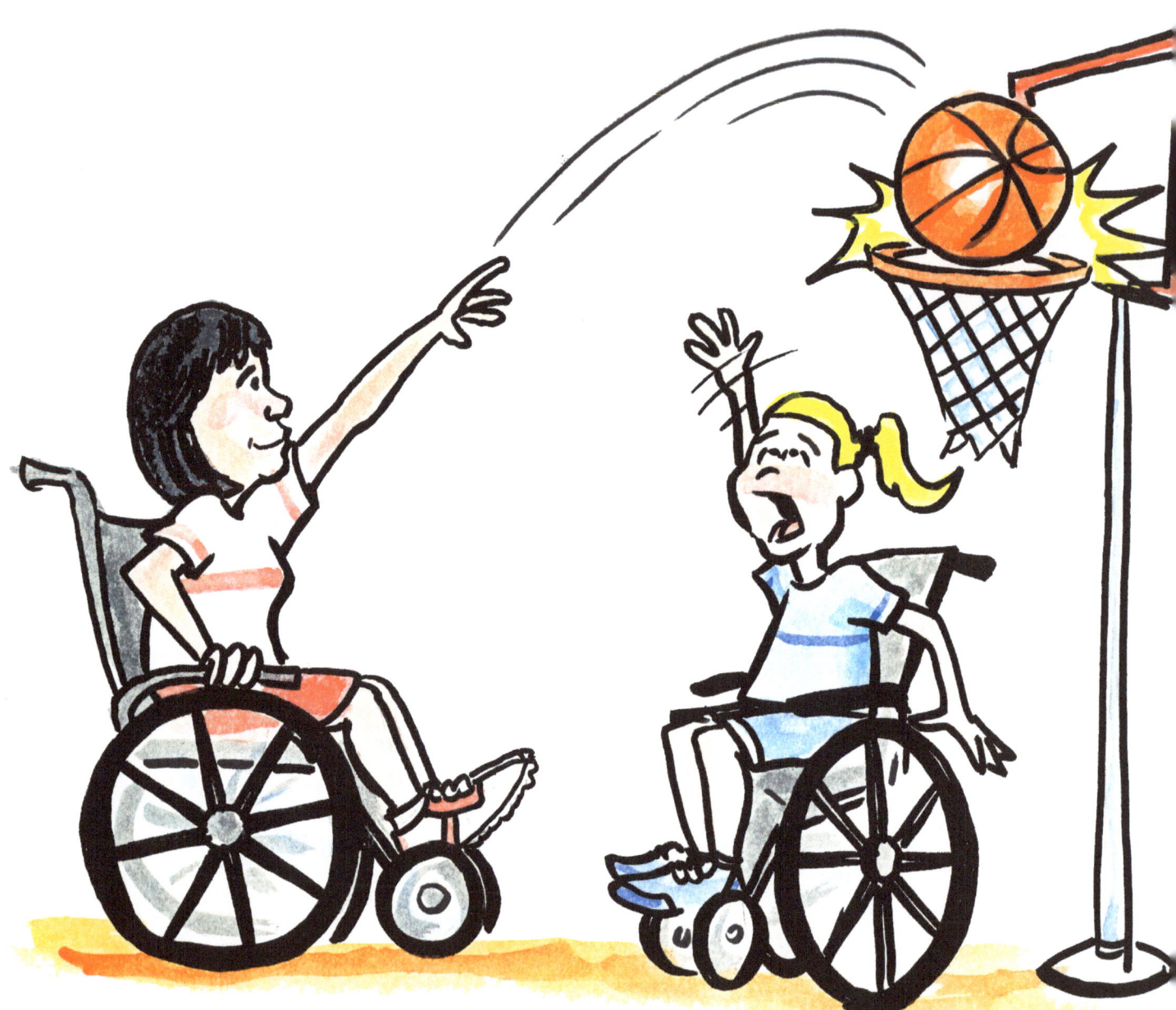

The next day we picked up Katherine.

We arrived at the large gym where Kelly plays wheelchair basketball. The other athletes were all in wheelchairs like Kelly and were warming up. "Wow, Aunt Manny there are sure a lot of people with cerebral palsy". Kelly was on fire that day and made 23 shots in a row. Katherine's eyes were wide with wonder. "Wow," Katherine said, "I couldn't do that!"

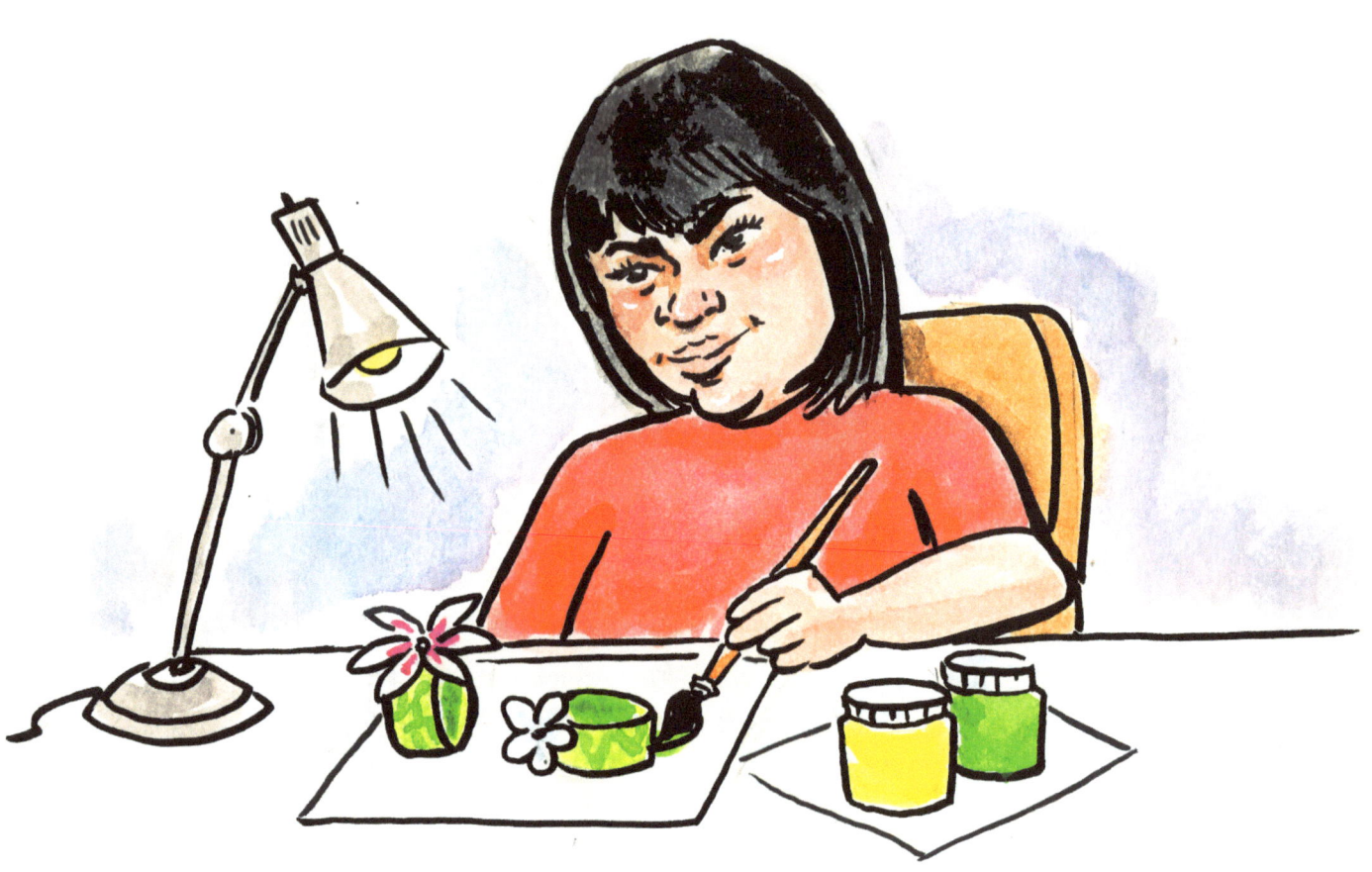

The following weekend we went to visit Katherine and Kelly brought her handmade one of a kind napkin rings to show Katherine. "How did Kelly do that?" "She paints the rings with her left hand and I help her with the hot glue gun and she puts on the decorations." "Wow, said Katherine these are really nice!"

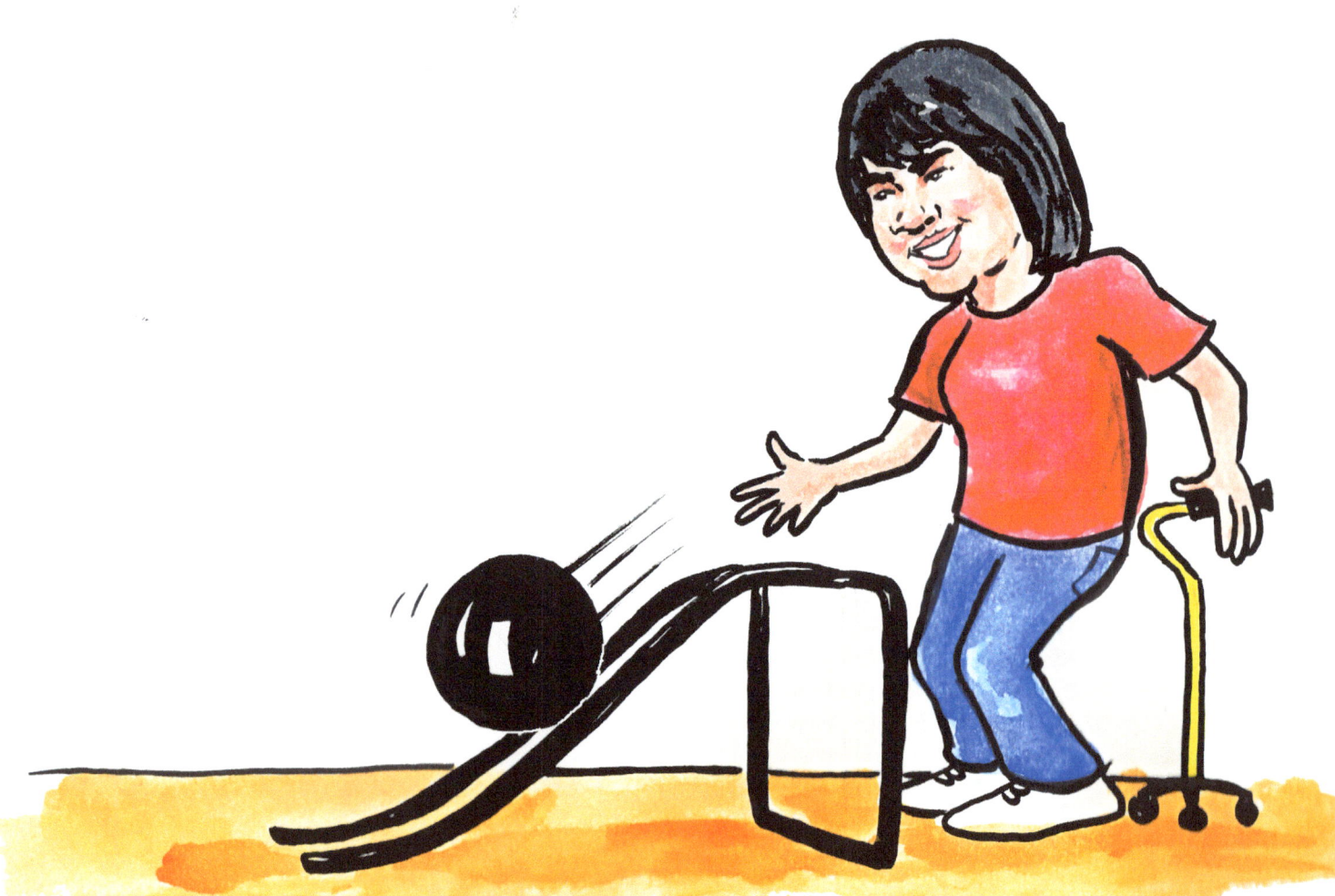

As soon as Katherine got in the car she asked "Can I help Kelly learn to write like me?" "No Katherine Kelly writes her name her way. It looks different from how you write your name, but it's her way." She asked if she could help Kelly learn to read and I said Kelly looks at the pictures. She can tell a story, maybe not like the words that are written, but it's her way. We took Katherine to watch Kelly bowl. Kelly uses a ramp for the ball. "Aunt Manny why does Kelly use the ramp to bowl?" "Kelly bowls in a different way. She uses the ramp to help steady the ball so she can push it with all her might!" Kelly got a 132 and no gutter balls. "Wow, Katherine said, I couldn't do that!"

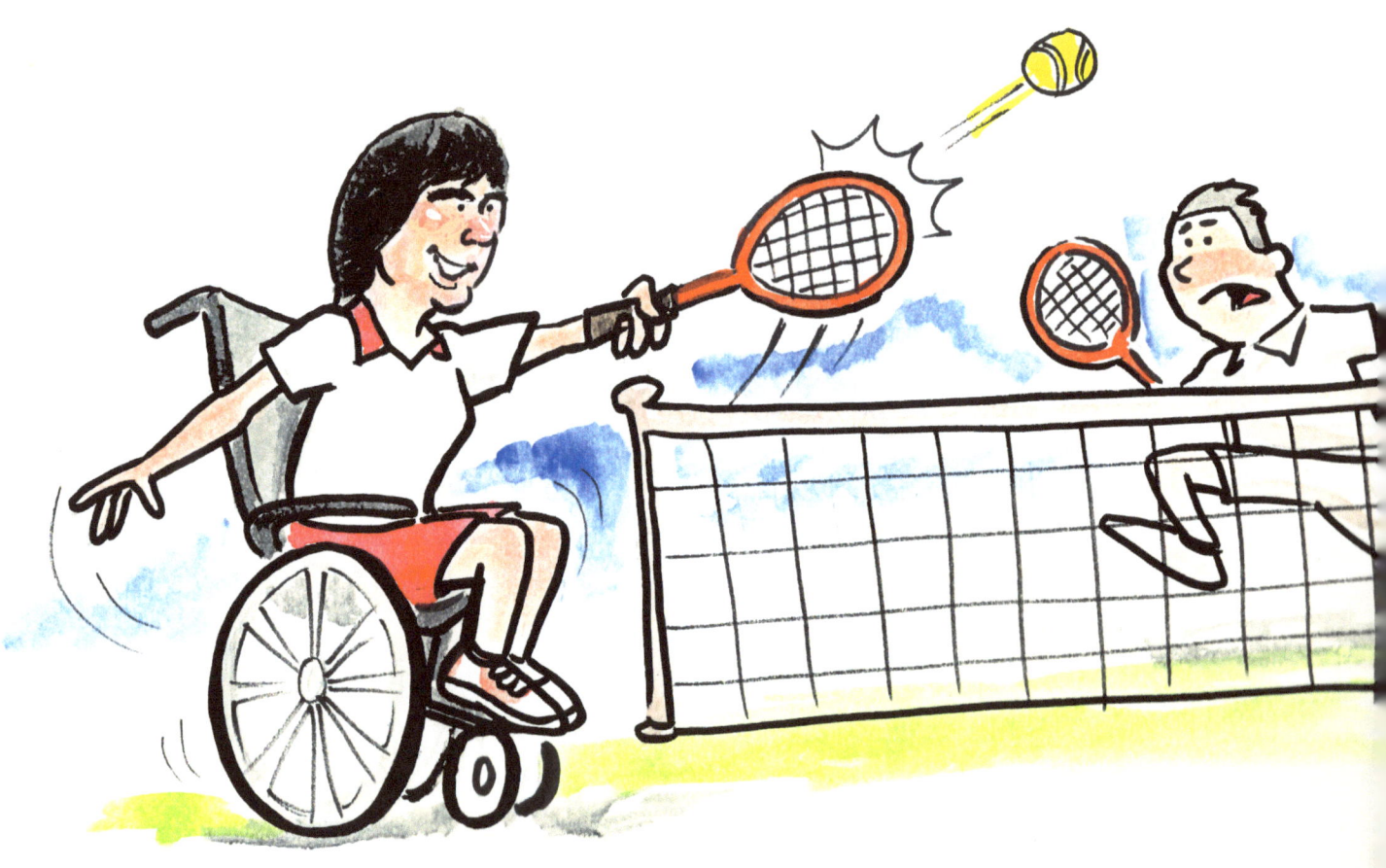

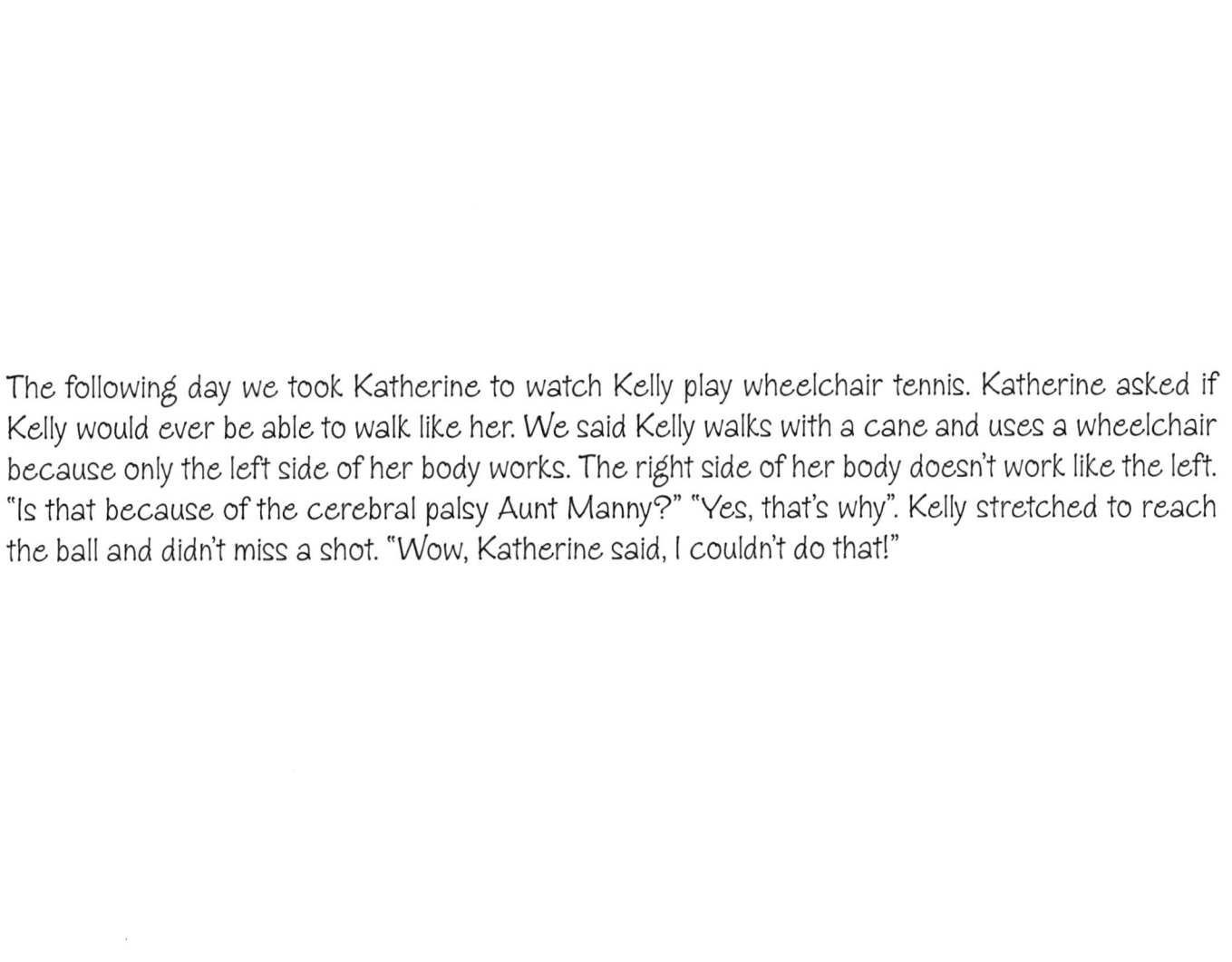

The following day we took Katherine to watch Kelly play wheelchair tennis. Katherine asked if Kelly would ever be able to walk like her. We said Kelly walks with a cane and uses a wheelchair because only the left side of her body works. The right side of her body doesn't work like the left. "Is that because of the cerebral palsy Aunt Manny?" "Yes, that's why". Kelly stretched to reach the ball and didn't miss a shot. "Wow, Katherine said, I couldn't do that!"

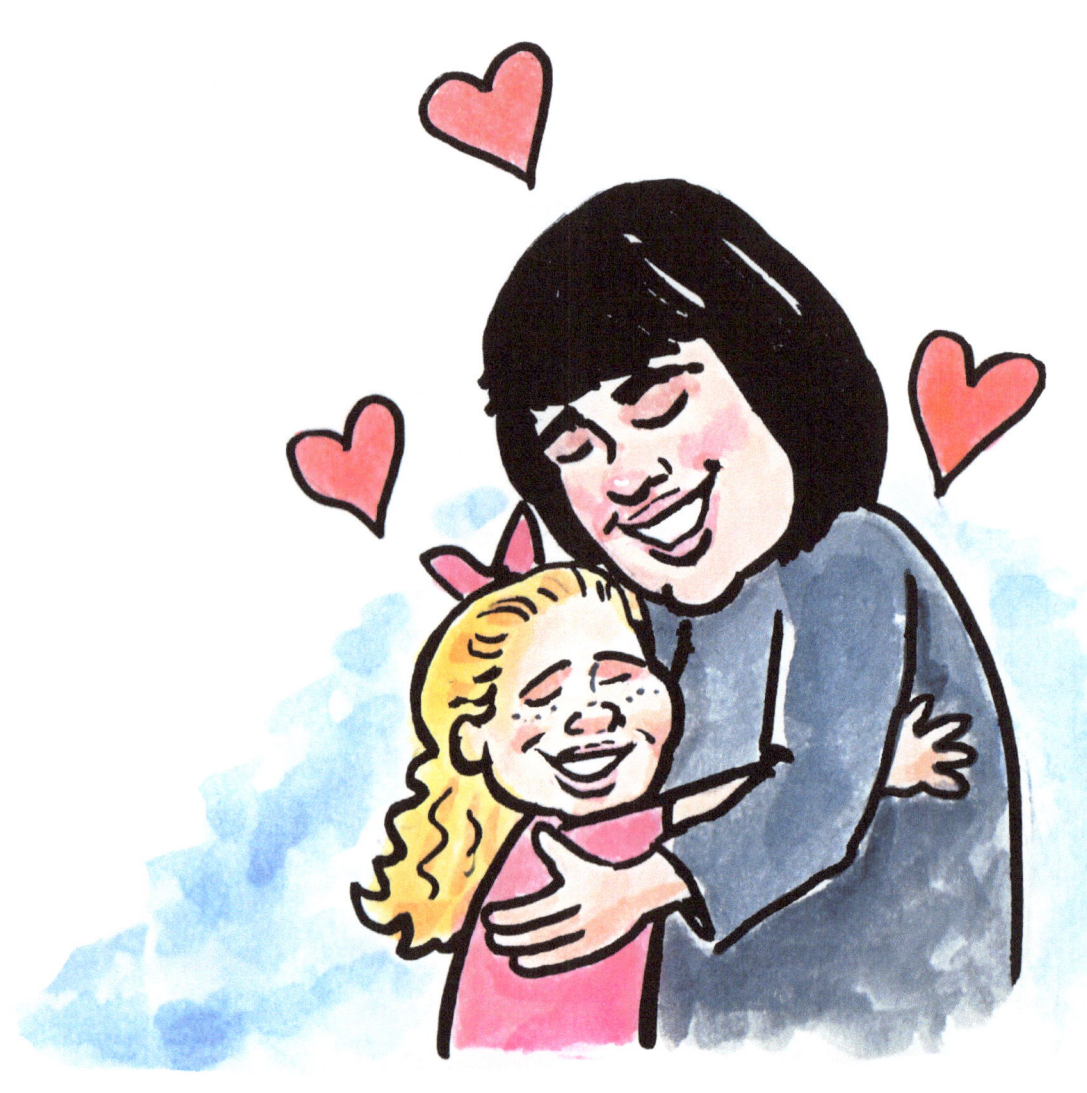

Katherine asked if Kelly will ever get married and have children. "Gee Katherine I don't know. Kelly is a beautiful woman and she has lots of love in her heart. She has cerebral palsy which makes her do things differently, who knows; maybe she'll have a different kind of marriage some day." Katherine thought about that. And with the innocence of a 6 year old and her new found knowledge asked, "Aunt Manny, I really want to help Kelly, what CAN I do?" Before we had time to answer Katherine blurted out—"I can help her make the napkin rings and we can sell them in a store and people can buy them and see what Kelly, who has cerebral palsy can do!"

www.ingramcontent.com/pod-product-compliance
Lightning Source LLC
Chambersburg PA
CBHW060828290526
45792CB00005BB/1839